MORNING PILATES FOR PROFESSIONALS

Revitalize Your Day with Pilates as experts

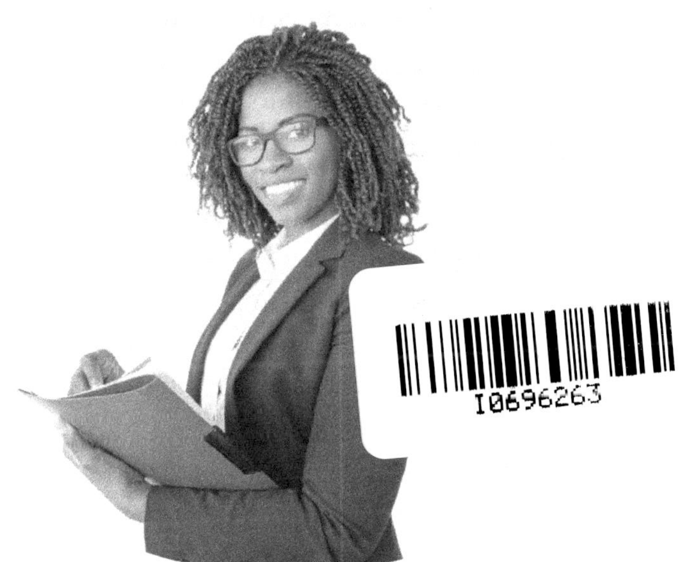

Lawrence R. Hale

Table of contents

INTRODUCTION 5

.... 5

Chapter 1: 6

An overview of Pilates and its benefits for professionals.
.... 6

The importance of starting your day with a mindful and
fitness-oriented routine. 8

Chapter 2: 10

The Science behind Morning Exercise 10

Chapter 3: 12

Setting Up Your Morning Pilates Space 12

Chapter 4: 14

Breathing Techniques in Morning Pilates 14

Chapter 5 16

A 30-Day Morning Pilates Challenge 16

30 days morning Pilates exercises for professionals 18

Chapter 6 23

Building a Strong Foundation 23

Chapter 7 24

Chapter 8 26

Stress Reduction through Morning Pilates 26

How Pilates can help manage stress and anxiety 28

Mindfulness techniques to incorporate into your routine.
.... 28

Chapter 9 29

Nutrition and Morning Pilates 29

The role of nutrition in optimizing morning Pilates performance. 31

Pre- and post-workout meal ideas for professionals. 31

Chapter 10 34

Sustainable Morning Pilates Habits 34

Tips for making morning Pilates a long-term habit. 35

Balancing Pilates with a busy professional schedule.... 36

CONCLUSION 38

INTRODUCTION

Pilates is a popular and highly effective form of exercise that has gained recognition worldwide for its numerous physical and mental health benefits. Originally developed by Joseph Pilates in the early 20th century, it has evolved into a comprehensive system of movements that improve strength, flexibility, balance, and overall well-being. For professionals in various fields, Pilates offers a range of advantages that can significantly enhance their physical health and mental resilience.

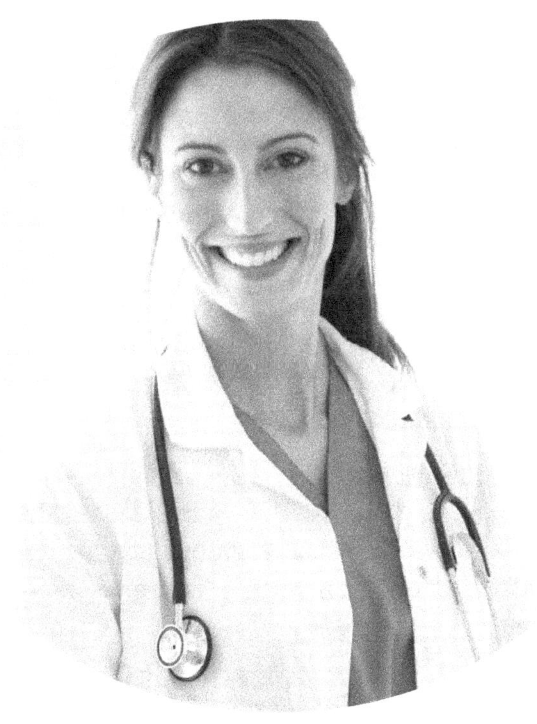

An overview of Pilates and its benefits for professionals.

Benefits of Pilates for Professionals:

Improved Posture: Pilates helps individuals develop better posture by strengthening the muscles responsible for supporting the spine. This can be especially beneficial for professionals who spend long hours sitting at a desk or working on a computer.

Core Strength: A strong core is essential for maintaining stability and balance. Pilates specifically targets the core muscles, which can help professionals in various industries perform their tasks more efficiently and with less risk of injury.

Increased Flexibility: Pilates incorporates stretching exercises that enhance flexibility, making it easier for professionals to move comfortably and perform tasks that require bending and reaching.

Stress Reduction: The mindful and controlled breathing techniques used in Pilates can help reduce stress and promote relaxation. This can be particularly beneficial for professionals dealing with high-pressure work environments.

Enhanced Body Awareness: Pilates encourages practitioners to focus on body awareness and proper alignment. This awareness can translate into better ergonomics and injury prevention in the workplace.

Injury Prevention and Rehabilitation: Pilates is often recommended by physical therapists and healthcare professionals for injury prevention and rehabilitation. Professionals who have suffered injuries can use Pilates as a means of recovery and strengthening.

Increased Energy and Stamina: Regular Pilates practice can boost energy levels and improve stamina, helping professionals stay alert and focused throughout the workday.

Better Breathing: Pilates emphasizes controlled breathing techniques, which can lead to improved lung capacity and better oxygenation of the body. This can be especially valuable for professionals who use their voices extensively, such as public speakers or teachers.

Enhanced Mental Clarity: Pilates requires concentration and mental focus, which can sharpen cognitive skills and decision-making abilities. Professionals may find that their mental clarity improves with consistent practice.

Work-Life Balance: Pilates provides an opportunity for professionals to disconnect from the demands of work and engage in self-care. It promotes a healthier work-life balance by encouraging regular exercise and stress relief.

1. Boosts Physical Health:

Engaging in a fitness-oriented routine in the morning jumpstarts your metabolism, increasing blood flow and oxygen delivery to your muscles and organs.

Regular physical activity helps maintain a healthy weight, reduces the risk of chronic illnesses like heart disease and diabetes, and improves overall cardiovascular health.

2. Enhances Mental Well-being: Mindfulness exercises, such as meditation or deep breathing, can reduce stress, anxiety, and depressive symptoms. Exercise releases endorphins, which are natural mood lifters, promoting a positive outlook and better emotional resilience.

3. Increases Productivity: A mindful routine can help you clear your mind, set clear intentions, and prioritize tasks for the day. This can lead to a better result and time management. Also Physical activity has been shown to enhance cognitive function, memory, and problem-solving skills, making you more efficient in your professional and personal life.

4. Encourages Consistency: Starting the day with a routine makes it more likely that you'll stick to healthy habits. It creates a structured and predictable start to your day.

Consistency is key to achieving long-term fitness and mindfulness goals, whether it's weight loss, muscle gain, or reduced stress.

5. Promotes Self-Care: Prioritizing your health and well-being at the beginning of the day sends a powerful message that self-care matters. It sets the tone for self-compassion and self-respect. Taking time for yourself in the morning can improve your self-esteem and overall sense of worth.

6. Improves Focus and Concentration: Mindfulness practices enhance your ability to stay present and focused, which can translate into better concentration at work or during important tasks. Exercise has been shown to increase attention span and cognitive flexibility, which can be invaluable in a professional setting.

7. Enhances Physical Fitness: A fitness-oriented morning routine helps you build and maintain physical strength, flexibility, and endurance. It can be easier to make exercise a habit when it's part of your daily morning routine, ensuring that you consistently work towards your fitness goals.

8. Sets a Positive Tone: A mindful and fitness-oriented start to your day can put you in a positive mindset, which can influence your interactions with others and the overall atmosphere of your day. It can be a source of motivation and a reminder of your commitment to self-improvement.

Chapter 2

The Science behind Morning Exercise

Morning exercise has a solid scientific foundation, offering a range of physical and mental health benefits that can significantly impact your overall well-being. Here's a glimpse into the science behind morning exercise:

1. Circadian Rhythms: Our bodies have internal clocks known as circadian rhythms that influence various physiological processes. Morning exercise aligns with these rhythms, as our body temperature, hormone levels, and cardiovascular function are optimized for physical activity during this time. This leads to enhanced exercise performance and reduced perceived effort.

2. Metabolism and Weight Management: Morning exercise can help regulate metabolism. It jumpstarts the metabolic rate, leading to increased calorie expenditure throughout the day. Moreover, it may help control appetite and reduce overall food intake, contributing to weight management and fat loss.

3. Stress Reduction: Exercise triggers the release of endorphins, neurotransmitters that act as natural mood lifters. Morning workouts help reduce cortisol, the stress hormone, which can lead to improved stress management and mental resilience.

4. Cognitive Function: Physical activity increases blood flow to the brain, improving cognitive function, memory, and attention. Morning exercise can enhance mental clarity, focus, and problem-solving abilities, making it an excellent choice for professionals.

5. Sleep Quality: Regular morning exercise has been linked to better sleep patterns. It helps regulate the sleep-wake cycle, improves sleep quality, and reduces the time it takes to fall asleep.

6. Consistency: Morning routines are often more consistent. By exercising in the morning, you're less likely to skip workouts due to schedule changes or fatigue that can accumulate throughout the day.

7. Hormone Regulation: Morning exercise can positively affect hormones such as insulin sensitivity and growth hormone secretion. This can lead to better glucose control, which is vital for long-term health.

8. Long-Term Health: Regular morning exercise is associated with a reduced risk of chronic diseases, including heart disease, diabetes, and certain types of cancer. It supports overall longevity and well-being.

Chapter 3

Setting Up Your Morning Pilates Space

Setting up a dedicated morning Pilates space in your home can make a world of difference in your daily routine. It not only encourages consistency but also creates a serene and motivating environment for your practice. Here's how to set up your morning Pilates space effectively:

1. Choose a Quiet and Well-Lit Area: Select a space that is quiet and receives natural light. This will create a calming atmosphere and make your morning practice more enjoyable.

2. Clear the Clutter: DE clutter the area to create a sense of tranquility. Remove any unnecessary items that may distract you from your Pilates routine.

3. Use a Comfortable Mat: Invest in a good-quality Pilates mat that provides cushioning and support for your exercises. A non-slip mat is essential for safety.

4. Accessorize Sparingly: While Pilates doesn't require much equipment, you may want to include items like resistance bands, small hand weights, or a Pilates ball. Keep them neatly stored nearby for easy access.

5. Consider Mirrors: Mirrors can help you check your form and alignment during exercises. Place a full-length mirror at a suitable angle

6. Play Relaxing Music: Soft, soothing music can enhance the ambiance of your Pilates space. You get to create a playlist with your favorite calming tunes.

7. Set up a Relaxation Corner: Include a small corner for relaxation with a comfortable chair or cushion where you can meditate or simply unwind after your Pilates session.

8. Keep it Personal: Personalize your space with items that motivate you, such as inspirational quotes, artwork, or plants. Ensure to make it a space you enjoy spending your time in.

9. Organize Storage: Have designated storage for your Pilates accessories and props to keep the space tidy and organized.

10. Commit to Consistency: Lastly, commit to using your Pilates space regularly. Consistency is key to reaping the benefits of Pilates and creating a morning routine that sets a positive tone for your day.

Therefore by creating a dedicated morning Pilates space that is inviting and comfortable, you'll be more inclined to stick to your practice and experience the physical and mental benefits it offers. It's an investment in your well-being and a way to prioritize self-care at the start of each day.

Creating a conducive environment for your morning Pilates routine.

The equipment you might need and how to use it effectively.

Chapter 4

Breathing Techniques in Morning Pilates

Breathing Techniques in Morning Pilates

Breathing is a fundamental element of Pilates that plays a crucial role in enhancing the mind-body connection and maximizing the benefits of your morning Pilates routine. Here's a brief overview of the significance of breathing techniques in morning Pilates:

Mindful Breath Control: Morning Pilates isn't just about physical movement; it's also an opportunity to cultivate mindfulness. Proper breathing techniques promote mental focus and awareness, helping you connect with your body's movements more effectively.

Engage the Core: In Pilates, the breath is coordinated with movement to engage the core muscles. As you exhale, you can engage your deep abdominal muscles, promoting stability and control. This enhances the effectiveness of exercises aimed at strengthening the core.

Controlled Exhalation: Pilates encourages controlled exhalation during the most challenging part of an exercise. For example, during a core-strengthening exercise like the Hundred, you exhale forcefully while maintaining a strong core, which intensifies the workout and builds abdominal strength.

Improved Oxygenation: Deep, rhythmic breathing in Pilates enhances oxygen flow to muscles, aiding in their function and reducing the risk of fatigue and cramping during your morning routine.

Stress Reduction: Focusing on your breath helps reduce stress and tension, making your morning Pilates session a calming and centering experience. It can even set a right positive tone for the rest of the day.

Enhanced Posture and Alignment: Proper breathing techniques in Pilates encourage good posture and alignment. As you breathe deeply and engage your core, you naturally improve your spinal alignment, which can alleviate back pain and discomfort.

Breath Awareness: Morning Pilates provides an opportunity to develop better breath awareness. This newfound awareness can carry over into your daily life, helping you manage stress and maintain better posture throughout the day.

Incorporating mindful breathing techniques into your morning Pilates practice can transform it into a holistic experience that benefits both body and mind. As you synchronize your breath with movement, you'll not only strengthen your core and improve your physical fitness but also nurture a sense of tranquility and balance to start your day on a positive note.

Chapter 5

A 30-Day Morning Pilates Challenge

Are you ready to kick start your mornings with a burst of energy, improved flexibility, and enhanced core strength? If so, the 30-Day Morning Pilates Challenge might be just the journey you need. This challenge offers a structured and manageable way to introduce the power of Pilates into your daily routine, setting the stage for a healthier and more invigorating lifestyle.

The Challenge: What is it? The 30-Day Morning Pilates Challenge is a commitment to incorporate a Pilates routine into the start of each day for an entire month. It typically involves a series of Pilates exercises, focusing on core strength, flexibility, and mindful breathing. Participants can choose to follow guided routines, enroll in online classes, or create their own tailored sessions.

The Benefits: Why Take the Challenge? Improved Physical Fitness: Morning Pilates sessions help build a strong and stable core, enhance flexibility, and improve overall muscle tone.

Boosted Energy: Engaging in exercise first thing in the morning increases blood flow and releases endorphins, providing a natural energy boost to kick start your day.

Enhanced Mental Clarity: The combination of movement and mindful breathing can sharpen focus, improve cognitive function, and reduce stress and anxiety.

Establishing Healthy Habits: The 30-day commitment encourages the formation of healthy habits, making it more likely to continue with a regular Pilates practice beyond the challenge.

Better Posture: Pilates emphasizes proper alignment and posture, which can alleviate back and neck pain associated with poor posture.

Personal Growth: The challenge offers an opportunity for self-discovery and personal growth as you push your physical and mental boundaries.

How to Get Started

Set Clear Goals: Define what you hope to achieve with the challenge. Whether it's increased flexibility, weight loss, or stress reduction, having specific goals can keep you motivated.

Create a Schedule: Determine the best time for your morning Pilates practice and stick to it. Consistency is the sole key to reaping the benefits.

Seek Guidance: Consider enrolling in online Pilates classes or using instructional videos to ensure you're performing exercises correctly.

Stay Accountable: Share your challenge with friends or join a Pilates community for support and accountability.

Listening to Your Body: Paying attention to your body's signals and languages if you need a rest day or modifications to the exercises, don't hesitate to make adjustments.

30-Day Morning Pilates Challenge is an opportunity for personal transformation. By dedicating just a portion of your morning to Pilates, you can experience significant improvements in physical fitness, mental well-being, and overall health. As you progress through the challenge, you'll not only witness positive changes in your body but also cultivate a sense of discipline and self-care that can extend well beyond the 30 days. So, are you up for the challenge?

Designing a month-long program to kick start your day with Pilates. Tracking your progress and staying motivated.

30 days morning Pilates exercises for professionals

Foundation Exercises (Day 1-10):

Pelvic Tilts:

Starting the Positioning: Lie down on your back with your knees bent and your feet flat on the floor.

Execution: Inhale to prepare, then exhale as you tilt your pelvis upward, pressing your lower back into the floor. Inhale to return to a neutral position. Focus on engaging your core muscles.

Repetitions: Perform 10 repetitions.

Single Leg Stretch:

Starting Position: Lie on your back with your knees bent and your feet lifted off the ground in a tabletop position.

Execution: Inhale to prepare, then exhale as you extend one leg while hugging the other knee toward your chest. Switch legs and repeat.   By keeping your core engaged and maintaining a stable pelvis.

Repetitions: Do 10 reps on each leg.

Double Leg Stretch: Starting Position: Lie on your back with both knees pulled into your chest.

Execution: Inhale to reach your arms and legs away from your body. Exhale as you return to the starting position by hugging your knees to your chest. Keep your core engaged throughout the movement.

Repetitions: Perform 10 reps.

Spine Stretch Forward: Starting Position: Sit with your legs extended, feet flexed, and your arms extended in front of you.

Execution: Inhale to sit tall, then exhale as you round your spine and reach forward with a flat back. Inhale to sit back up. Keep your core engaged and your shoulders relaxed.

Repetitions: Do 10 reps.

Swan Dive:

Starting Position: Lie face down with your arms extended overhead and your legs together.

Execution: Inhale as you lift your chest, arms, and legs off the floor, arching your back. Exhale as you lower back down. Focus on using your back muscles to lift, not your arms.

Repetitions: Perform 10 reps.

Intermediate Exercises (Day 11-20):

Rolling Like a Ball:

Starting Position: Sit with your knees pulled into your chest, feet off the ground, and arms around your shins.

Execution: Roll backward onto your upper back, then use your core strength to roll back up to the starting position without using your hands. Keep your feet off the ground throughout.

Repetitions: Do 10 reps.

Single Leg Circles:

Starting Position: Lie on your back with one leg extended up toward the ceiling and the other leg extended just above the ground.

Execution: Make small circles with the extended leg, controlling the movement with your core. Perform 10 reps in each direction (clockwise and counterclockwise) before switching legs.

Plank:

Starting Position: Beginning in a push-up way with your hands directly under your shoulders and ensuring your body in a straight line.

Execution: Hold this position, keeping your core engaged, your back flat, and your neck in line with your spine. Start with a 30-second hold and gradually increase the time as you progress.

Leg Pull Front:

Starting Position: Start in a plank position with your hands under your shoulders.

Execution: Lift one leg off the ground and reach it forward while maintaining a strong plank position. Alternate legs for 10 reps.

Saw: Starting Position: Sit with your legs wide apart, arms extended to the sides.

Execution: Rotate your upper body to one side, reaching your opposite hand toward the opposite foot, then return to the center and switch sides. Keep your legs grounded and your core engaged.

Repetitions: Perform 10 reps on each side.

Advanced Exercises (Day 21-30):

Teaser: Starting Position: Lie on your back with your legs extended.

Execution: Inhale as you sit up, lifting your legs and reaching your arms toward your feet. Breathe out as you roll back down with control. This type of exercise challenges your core strength and balance.

Repetitions: Do 10 reps.

The Hundred: Starting Position: Lie on your back with your legs lifted off the ground, and your head and shoulders off the mat.

Execution: Pump your arms up and down while inhaling for 5 counts and exhaling for 5 counts. Maintain a strong core throughout. Repeat for a total of hundred counts.

Boomerang:

Starting Position: Sit with your legs extended.

Execution: Roll backward, then roll back up, lifting your legs and rolling forward again. This type of exercise challenges your control and balance.

Repetitions: Perform 10 reps.

Corkscrew: Starting Position: Lie on your back with your legs extended straight up.

Execution: Circle your legs to one side, then back to the center, and over to the other side. Keep your core engaged to control the movement. Perform 10 reps.

Control Balance: Starting Position: Lie on your back with one leg extended up and the other leg bent.

Execution: Lift your torso and reach your arms toward your extended leg, then switch legs and repeat. This exercise challenges your core and balance.

Repetitions: Do 10 reps on each side.

These exercises are progressively more challenging, so it's essential to maintain proper form and technique to avoid injury. Additionally, it's recommended to warm up before starting your Pilates routine and cool down afterward with some gentle stretches. If you're new to Pilates or have any concerns, consider seeking guidance from a certified Pilates instructor to ensure you're performing the exercises correctly and safely

Chapter 6

Building a Strong Foundation

FOR PROFESSIONALS, mornings can be hectic, but dedicating time to morning Pilates is an investment in your physical and mental well-being. It sets a strong foundation for the day, enhancing core strength, posture, and mental clarity. By prioritizing a consistent Pilates practice, professionals can boost energy, reduce stress, and improve focus, making them more efficient and resilient in their work. It's not just exercise; it's a daily commitment to self-care that empowers professionals to tackle their challenges with confidence and vitality, ultimately leading to a more balanced and successful professional life.

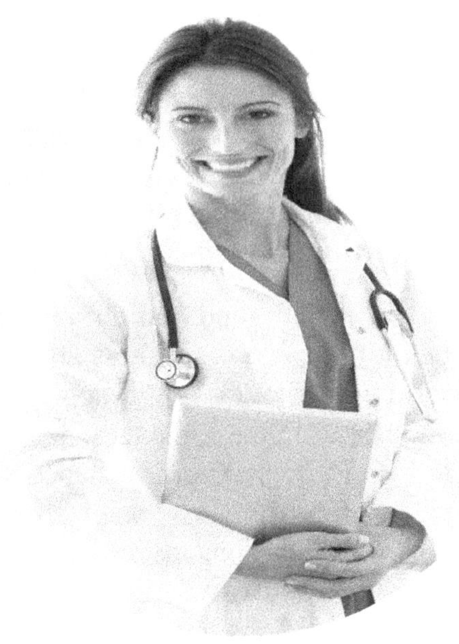

Chapter 7

Flexibility and Mobility

1. Flexibility: Flexibility refers to the range of motion in your joints and muscles. It's the ability of your body to move freely and easily through a full range of motion without experiencing discomfort or stiffness.

Morning Pilates helps improve flexibility by incorporating dynamic stretching exercises that lengthen and elongate muscles. This is essential for professionals who may spend long hours sitting or in sedentary positions, which can lead to muscle tightness and reduced flexibility. Enhanced flexibility can lead to better posture, reduced risk of injuries, and improved performance in daily activities and work-related tasks.

2. Mobility: Mobility is related to flexibility but focuses on the functional range of motion in your joints. It's not just about being able to stretch; it's about being able to move with control and stability. Morning Pilates emphasizes mobility through exercises that engage and strengthen muscles around the joints, promoting stability and balance.

Improved mobility is particularly valuable for professionals who need to move efficiently and comfortably throughout the day. It can help prevent joint stiffness and discomfort, especially in areas prone to tension, such as the neck, shoulders, and lower back. In the context of morning Pilates, professionals can benefit greatly from enhanced flexibility and mobility. These improvements can lead to reduced muscle tension, better posture, increased energy levels, and an overall sense of physical well-being. Incorporating regular morning Pilates sessions into your routine can help you maintain and continually improve your flexibility and mobility, ensuring you're prepared to face the demands of your professional life with comfort and confidence. Exploring Pilates exercises that enhance flexibility and mobility.

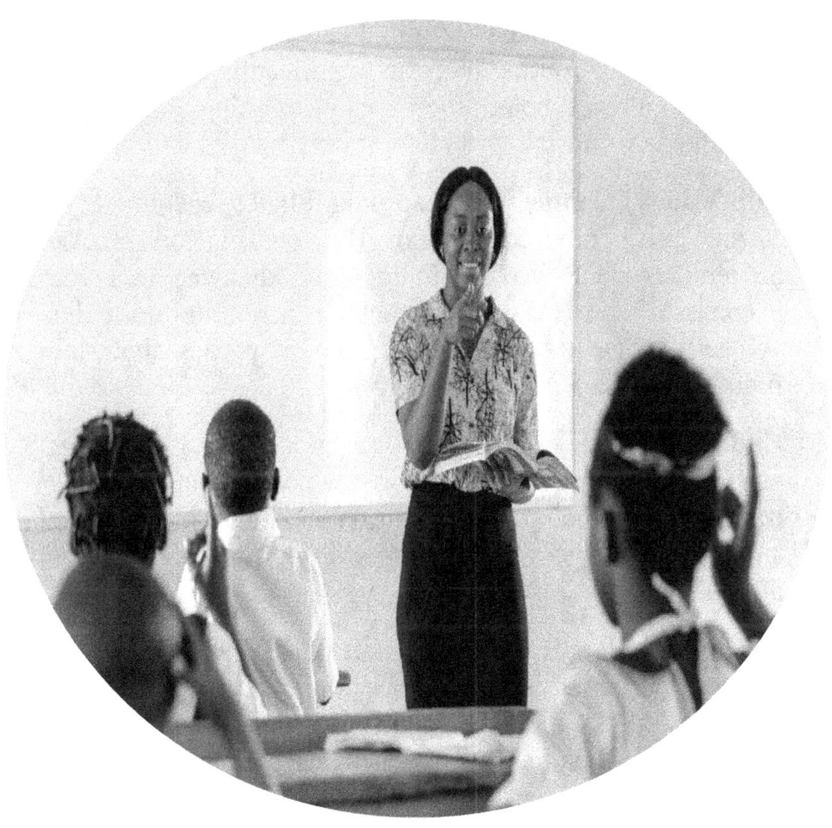

Chapter 8

Stress Reduction through Morning Pilates

Stress reduction through morning Pilates is a valuable aspect of this exercise routine that can significantly contribute to your overall well-being. Here's how morning Pilates can help alleviate stress:

Mind-Body Connection: Morning Pilates encourages a strong mind-body connection. By focusing on precise movements, controlled breathing, and body awareness, you become fully present in the moment. This mindfulness helps you let go of stressors from the past or worries about the future, promoting a sense of calm.

Endorphin Release: Like any form of exercise, Pilates prompts the release of endorphins, which are natural mood lifters. These "feel-good" chemicals can help reduce stress, anxiety, and depression, leaving you with a more positive outlook on your day.

Muscle Tension Relief: Stress often manifests as muscle tension, particularly in the neck, shoulders, and back. Morning Pilates includes stretching exercises that target these areas, helping to release tension and promote relaxation.

Stress Hormone Regulation: Engaging in physical activity, including Pilates, helps regulate stress hormones like cortisol. Consistent morning Pilates practice can lead to more balanced hormone levels, reducing the body's stress response.

Enhanced Sleep Quality: Stress can disrupt sleep patterns, leading to poor sleep quality. Regular morning Pilates can promote better sleep by reducing stress and anxiety, making it easier to fall asleep and stay asleep.

Improved Coping Mechanisms: As you progress in your Pilates practice, you develop better coping mechanisms for dealing with stress. You learn to manage discomfort during challenging exercises, which can translate into better stress management in other aspects of life.

Structured Routine: A morning Pilates routine provides structure to your day. Having a set time for self-care and exercise can reduce stress associated with a lack of routine or feeling overwhelmed by daily responsibilities.

Time for Self-Care: Prioritizing morning Pilates is an act of self-care. It sends a message to yourself that your well-being is essential, fostering a positive relationship with yourself and reducing stress associated with neglecting self-care.

How Pilates can help manage stress and anxiety.

Pilates is a powerful tool for managing stress and anxiety. Through its mindful movement and controlled breathing, Pilates cultivates a sense of calm and presence. The practice releases endorphins, natural mood boosters that counteract stress hormones. It also targets muscle tension, a common physical manifestation of stress. As you focus on proper alignment and posture, Pilates reduces the strain caused by poor posture, alleviating pain associated with stress. Enhanced cognitive function and improved sleep quality further contribute to stress and anxiety management. Pilates empowers individuals to take control of their well-being, providing both physical and mental relief from the challenges of daily life.

Mindfulness techniques to incorporate into your routine.

Mindfulness techniques are invaluable for promoting mental well-being and reducing stress in our fast-paced lives. Incorporating these practices into your daily routine can enhance your overall sense of calm and presence. Begin by setting aside a few minutes each day for mindful breathing exercises. Stay focused on your breath while inhaling and exhaling deeply. Another technique is body scanning, where you mentally explore each part of your body, releasing tension as you go. Mindful walking or eating can also be transformative, engaging your senses fully in the moment. These simple yet powerful techniques offer a pathway to greater mindfulness and a more balanced, peaceful existence.

Chapter 9

Nutrition and Morning Pilates

NUTRITION plays a crucial role in supporting your morning Pilates routine and optimizing its benefits. Here's what you should know about the relationship between nutrition and morning Pilates:

Pre-Exercise Nutrition: Eating a light and balanced meal or snack before your morning Pilates session can provide you with the energy and stamina needed for your workout. Opt for easily digestible options, such as a banana, yogurt, or a small serving of oatmeal, about 30 minutes to an hour before your session.

Stay Hydrated: Hydration is key to any exercise routine, including Pilates. Drink a glass of water when you wake up to rehydrate after the night's rest. Staying hydrated throughout the day is essential to prevent fatigue and muscle cramps during your session.

Post-Exercise Nutrition: After your morning Pilates session, aim to refuel with a balanced meal that includes a combination of carbohydrates and protein. This will help with the muscle recovery and replenishing energy stores. For example, a vegetable omelet with whole-grain toast or a smoothie with protein powder and fruits can be excellent choices.

Avoid Heavy Meals: While it's important to eat before and after your session, avoid heavy, greasy, or high-fiber meals right before Pilates, as they can lead to discomfort during exercise.

Listening to Your Body: By paying attention to your body's hunger and fullness cues. Everybody's nutritional needs are different, so it's essential to find what works best for you.

Balanced Diet: Maintaining a well-balanced diet overall is crucial for your energy levels and overall health, which in turn supports your morning Pilates practice. Ensure that your diets which includes a variety of nutrient-rich foods, including fruits and vegetable with lean proteins, whole grains, and healthy fats.

Supplements: Some individuals may benefit from supplements like B-vitamins, magnesium, or iron if they have specific deficiencies that affect their energy levels. It is advisable you consult with a healthcare professional before adding supplements to your routine.

Timing Matters: Try to time your meals and snacks to provide a steady source of energy throughout the day. Small, frequent meals can help stabilize blood sugar levels and sustain your energy levels.

It is very important to note that proper nutrition plays a significant role in your ability to perform well during morning Pilates sessions. It provides the energy and nutrients necessary for muscle function and recovery. By adopting a balanced diet and being mindful of your food choices before and after your Pilates practice, you can enhance the overall effectiveness of your workouts and promote better health and well-being.

NUTRITION is a vital component in unlocking the full potential of your morning Pilates practice. To optimize performance, consider your fuel. A light, balanced pre-Pilates snack, like yogurt or a banana, boosts energy. Post-workout, focus on a balanced meal with carbohydrates and protein to aid muscle recovery. Staying hydrated is equally important. Proper nutrition ensures you have the stamina, endurance, and muscle support to engage fully in your Pilates routine. It's the key to maximizing the benefits of your morning sessions, leaving you refreshed, revitalized, and ready to face the day with vigor.

Pre- and post-workout meal ideas for professionals.

Pre-Workout Meal Ideas for Professionals:

Banana and Almond Butter: This quick and easy snack provides a balance of carbohydrates, healthy fats, and protein, offering sustained energy for your workout.

Greek Yogurt with Berries and Honey: Greek yogurt is rich in protein, and the berries provide natural sugars for a quick energy boost. Drizzle with honey for added flavor.

Oatmeal with Nuts and Fruit: A bowl of oatmeal topped with chopped nuts and fresh fruit is an excellent source of complex carbohydrates, fiber, and healthy fats to fuel your workout.

Whole-Grain Toast with Avocado: Avocado offers healthy fats, while whole-grain toast provides complex carbohydrates. This type of combination keeps you full and energized.

Smoothie: Blend spinach, banana, almond milk, and a scoop of protein powder for a nutrient-packed, portable pre-workout meal.

Post-Workout Meal Ideas for Professionals:

Grilled Chicken Salad: A chicken salad with leafy greens and a variety of colorful vegetables provides protein for muscle recovery and essential nutrients.

Quinoa and Vegetable Stir-Fry: Quinoa is a complete protein, and a stir-fry with plenty of veggies offers a balanced post-workout meal.

Salmon with Sweet Potatoes: Salmon is rich in omega-3 fatty acids, while sweet potatoes provide complex carbohydrates. This combo aids muscle repair and glycogen replenishment.

Egg and Vegetable Scramble: Scrambled eggs with a mix of vegetables like peppers, spinach, and tomatoes is a protein-packed option that supports muscle recovery.

Protein-Packed Smoothie: Blend a protein powder with almond milk, frozen berries, and a handful of spinach for a quick and convenient post-workout meal.

Whole-Grain Wrap with Turkey: A whole-grain wrap filled with lean turkey, hummus, and plenty of veggies is an excellent source of protein, fiber, and vitamins.

Cottage Cheese with Pineapple: Cottage cheese is high in protein, and pineapple adds natural sweetness and vitamins for muscle recovery it is important to remember to stay hydrated by drinking more water before, during, and after your workout. These meal ideas for professionals can help you stay energized, recover efficiently, and perform at your best throughout your busy day.

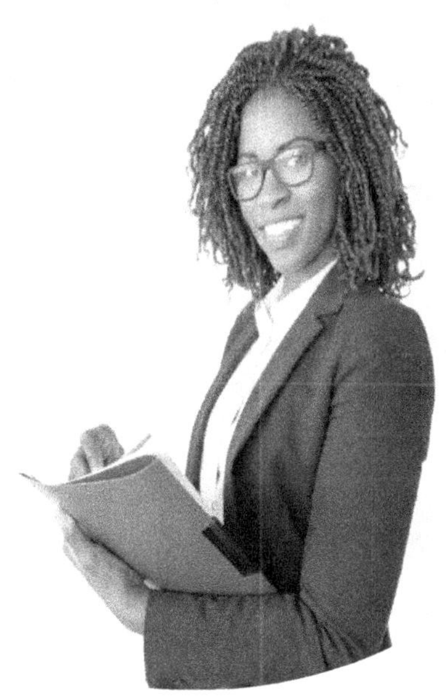

Chapter 10

Sustainable Morning Pilates Habits

Sustainable morning Pilates habits are not only beneficial for your physical and mental well-being but also for the environment and long-term commitment to a healthy lifestyle. Here's why they matter:

1. Consistency: Sustainable habits are built on consistency. By making Pilates a regular part of your morning routine, you ensure that it becomes a lifelong practice, reaping the continuous benefits of improved strength, flexibility, and mental clarity.

2. Eco-Friendly Choices: Consider eco-friendly options in your Pilates practice, such as using a non-toxic, biodegradable mat and practicing outdoors when possible. This reduces your environmental footprint while enhancing your connection with nature.

3. Mindful Eating: Sustainable Pilates habits extend to your nutrition. Choose whole, locally sourced, and minimally processed foods that support your energy needs and overall health.

4. Quality Sleep: Prioritize quality sleep to support your morning Pilates routine. A well-rested body and mind are better equipped to perform and recover.5. Mental Health: Sustainable habits foster mental well-being. Pilates promotes mindfulness, helping you manage stress and anxiety while maintaining a positive outlook on life.

6. Injury Prevention: Consistency in Pilates leads to better muscle and joint health, reducing the risk of injuries and enhancing your ability to engage in physical activity throughout your life.

Sustainable morning Pilates habits not only benefit you but also contribute to a healthier planet and a more balanced and fulfilling lifestyle. They serve as a foundation for lifelong well-being and vitality, ensuring you can enjoy the benefits of Pilates for years to come.

Tips for making morning Pilates a long-term habit.

Creating a long-term morning Pilates habit involves consistency and commitment. The following tips are tips to make it stick:

Set a Routine: Designate a specific time for your morning Pilates. Consistency builds habit.

Start Slow: Begin with shorter sessions and gradually increase intensity and duration to prevent burnout.

Accountability: Partner with a friend or join a Pilates class to stay motivated and accountable.

Variety: Keep your routine fresh by trying different Pilates workouts and exercises.

Mindful Choice: Remember how Pilates benefits your body and mind, reinforcing your commitment.

Track Progress: Document your journey to see improvements and stay motivated.

Adaptability: Be flexible with your routine to accommodate life's changes while staying committed to your Pilates practice.

By simply implementing and incorporating these strategies into your daily life, morning Pilates can become a lasting and rewarding habit

Balancing Pilates with a busy professional schedule.

Balancing Pilates with a hectic professional schedule can be challenging but is entirely feasible with a strategic approach to time management and self-care. Below are some practical tips to help you achieve that balance

Schedule with Purpose: Treat your Pilates sessions as non-negotiable appointments. Block out dedicated time slots on your calendar and prioritize them like you would any work commitment.

Short and Effective Workouts: On busy days, opt for shorter, high-intensity Pilates workouts. Even a 15-20 minute session can provide significant benefits in terms of strength, flexibility, and mental clarity.

Early Morning Routine: Consider incorporating Pilates into your morning routine. It can help kick start your day with energy and focus. Set your alarm a bit earlier to create space for your practice.

Lunch Break Pilates: If your schedule allows, use your lunch break for a quick Pilates session. Many online platforms offer short Pilates workouts designed to fit into tight schedules.

Blend Work and Exercise: Explore creative ways to integrate Pilates into your workday. For instance, you can do seated leg stretches or gentle spinal twists at your desk to alleviate tension and promote flexibility.

Weekend Dedication: If weekdays are too packed, commit to longer Pilates sessions on the weekends. This can compensate for shorter workouts during the week.

Online and On-Demand Classes: Take advantage of online Pilates classes and on-demand videos. They offer flexibility in terms of timing and can be tailored to your schedule.

Stay Consistent: Consistency is key. Even if you can't practice Pilates every day, aim for regularity in your routine. Set achievable goals that align with your professional commitments.

Plan and Prep: Plan your Pilates sessions in advance and prepare your workout space to minimize setup time. This will help you maximize the efficiency of your practice.

Mindful Self-Care: Remember that Pilates is not just about physical exercise but also mental well-being. Use your Pilates sessions as a form of self-care, providing stress relief and mental clarity in the midst of a busy schedule.

Balancing Pilates with a busy professional life requires dedication and smart time management. By making your Pilates practice a priority and creatively fitting it into your schedule, you can enjoy the physical and mental benefits of Pilates while effectively managing your work commitments.

CONCLUSION

Morning Pilates for PROFESSIONALS is not merely a fitness routine; it is a transformative daily practice that empowers you to take charge of your physical and mental well-being. As you rise with the sun and embark on your Pilates journey, you are setting a powerful intention for the day ahead. You are strengthening your core, enhancing flexibility, and nurturing mindfulness, equipping yourself to face the challenges of your professional life with resilience and grace.

Morning Pilates offers you the gift of self-care, providing a sacred space to connect with your body, release stress, and cultivate a sense of calm in our fast-paced world. It is an investment in yourself, in your health, and in your future success.

So, rise and shine, dear **Professional,** and embrace the potential of each morning with Pilates. Whether it's the gentle stretch of a sunrise routine or the invigoration of a high-energy workout, this practice is your daily reminder that you are worth the time and effort it takes to be your best self. Make it a habit, and watch as the benefits ripple through your life, transforming not only your mornings but your entire professional journey. Your body, your mind, and your career will thank you for it.

Happy reading!